# OUR FAULT

### The infant mortality rate and the black community

### By Stanley G Buford, Ph.D.

*"Fool me once shame on you, fool me twice, shame on me!"*

*Mothers: If your Pediatrician/Family Doctor is not familiar with the tenents of this book with a view to concerns of the Black Family regarding the Medical Community; find another one!*

### Foreword By

### Junaid Khan M. D.

Dissertation:

Our Fault: The Infant Mortality Rate and the Black Community

"Countering the Effects of the Infant Mortality Rate for African American Women"

Presented to:

Apostle Dr. Sylvester P. Brinson III

Provost

Richard Daniel Henton University

President

Apostle Dr. Mark A. Henton

By Stanley G. Buford

Presented in fulfillment of the degree of:

Doctor of Philosophy in Christian Education and Leadership

# COPYRIGHT

**Our Fault: The Infant Mortality Rate and the Black Community**

TriDreams Productions

**Copyright © 2021 by Stanley G. Buford**

**Buford, Stanley G**

This publication is designed to provide accurate and authoritative information regarding the subject matter covered. It is sold under the understanding that the publisher is not engaged in rendering legal, accounting, or other professional services. If legal advice or other expert assistance is required, the services of a competent professional person should be sought.

*It's an Ebook, it's an Audiobook, it's a fantastic song; TriDreams Productions and you won't go wrong!* ®

**The Infant Mortality Rate and the Black Community**

**"Countering the effects of the Infant Mortality Rate for African American Women."**

Mr. Stanley G Buford's work by way of examination at Richard Daniel Henton University is really interesting and impressive relative to the infant mortality rate for African American women. He seems to have made connections with this research and put forth some recommendations. His recommendation has given a hand, via extensive study; to eliminate noted disparities and provided great suggestions to enhance the health of the African American community; specifically, Black women and infants, this work will go a long way to stem the tide of neglect and reduce the count of deaths that happen within the first year of life per one thousand live births in the African American community. Bravo!

*Shereef Abo Asy, M.D.*

*Family Practice*

# DEDICATION

Dedicated to all the hard-working families that make books like "Our Fault" possible

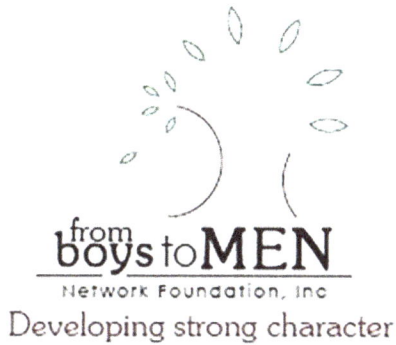

from
boys to MEN
Network Foundation, Inc
Developing strong character

Proceeds from this book will go to the From Boys to Men Network

A 501(C) (3) Non-Profit Foundation

Stanley G. Buford, Executive Director
7115 West North Avenue
Suite 163
Oak Park, IL 60302

fromboystomen@gmail.com

# FOREWORD

## By Junaid Khan, M. D.

A country's critical development is measured by the protection provided to the health of a mother and her child. By many accounts, the US is a developed state, but it holds the worst record of infant and maternal mortality compared to other developed countries. There is three times more chance of women dying in the US after giving birth than in Canada. The infant mortality rate is 76 percent high compared to other nations. If this data is divided by race, it is found that there is a higher rate of maternal and infant mortality among African American women than any other race.

I, Dr. Junaid khan, being a doctor, can say that black women and their babies die at an alarming rate compared to their counterparts. African American women not only face discrimination in other areas but in the health care profession also. The mistreatment that black women face during their appointments as well as after birth is shameful. Their concerns are ignored, which leads to a lot of stress. This stress then causes other pregnancy and birth-related issues. In 2017 the infant mortality rate of African American women was 10.97 percent, twice more than white, Asian, and Hispanic women.

A 27 years old activist and Black Lives Matter icon, Erica Garner, suffered her first heart attack shortly after giving birth.

Four months later, she suffered another heart attack which put her into a coma, and then she died while in that coma. Serena Williams, a famous tennis star, nearly died from postpartum complications. These two stories are not the only ones. These stories highlight the devastating problem in the US: those African American women are dying 3 to 4 times the rate of other women, and infants of black women are dying at twice the rate of other infants.

**"In addition to giving us key information about maternal and infant health, the infant mortality rate is an important marker of the overall health of a society."**

It does not matter if the black woman is rich or poor; the mistreatment of a pregnant black woman is everywhere in the US. Their concerns and complications are not only ignored, but one-quarter of black women report abuse and disrespect by health care professionals. These problems are just the tip of the iceberg of medical racism that black women face.

Research shows that providing proper treatment to pregnant women before, during, and after birth can significantly reduce the rate of infant mortality in the US. The majority of pregnancy-related deaths are preventable if health care professionals are loyal to their profession and do not indulge in discrimination. Any real change will require more research into why African American women have high infant mortality rates in the US.

I applaud Stanley G Buford's research through his doctoral dissertation at Richard Daniel Henton University. African American women and their babies can be saved if this research work is adhered to and implemented by stakeholders. Great political efforts are also required to undo racism in the US, which is undoubtedly a contributing factor in infant and maternal mortality rates. Racism's harmful effects cannot be ignored in infant and maternal health. African American women deserve better. Once racism is solved, health programs, counseling, and other solutions can be developed to reduce the rate of infant mortality, and thanks to Stanley G Buford's research, I can say, "let the healing begin."

# ACKNOWLEDGMENTS

I would like to give a huge thank you to everyone who has contributed towards the process of completing this research. A special mention goes my pastor, Dr. Apostle Mark Anthony Henton. A tremendous shout out to my dissertation supervisor, Dr. Apostle Sylvester Paul Brinson III. The support, guidance, advice and continuous encouragement throughout completing this process is really appreciated. I could not have asked for a better pastor or supervisor in helping me with publication of this dissertation/research. I would also like to thank my family for the Spiritual guidance and support provided throughout this endeavor.

A special thank you to my church family as they assisted with many theology studies that address discrepancies between the findings of traditional science/medicine and the teachings of the Bible.

Finally, thanks to my mother, Juanita Buford-Puckett, who at every step of my educational journey with a view to graduation from kindergarten through graduate school, would say: *"Congratulations, education is important and it is something no one can ever take away from you!"*

# Abstract: Our Fault: The Infant Mortality Rate and the Black Community

"Countering the effects of the Infant Mortality Rate for African American Women"

By Stanley G Buford

Richard Daniel Henton University

There is an indisputable truth in America: that black mothers, and their babies, die at a staggering rate during childbirth. When compared to their white counterparts, even across class lines, the difference is shocking.

Invariably during their prenatal appointments, black women are treated unbelievably poorly. Their concerns are ignored and minimized by doctors; medical staff treat them rudely; not to mention the institutionalized, systemic racism that black people in general endure throughout American society, which, for black women, is compounded by experiences of sexism. This research seeks to address and rectify this issue urging participants, from a biblical perspective:

1. Seek out community organizations which work to support black mothers in their respective state.

2. Make a conscious effort to advocate for themselves during medical appointments.

3. Practice some biblical based relaxation techniques to decrease their stress levels.

My hope as a male parent, and product of a mother who birthed 10 healthy children into the world, is that this research will provide the reader with some much-needed information on the current infant mortality crisis in America. My message to mothers from all walks of life is this: Remember that they deserve the best medical care possible, and sadly, that they may have to be very vocal in order to receive it. ***Our Fault: The Infant Mortality Rate and the Black Community;*** will delve deeper than other works previously with statistics and facts that ruminate, admonishing mothers to always seek out resources in their local communities first, stand up for themselves, and try their best to reduce stress levels through things like prayer, meditation and thanksgiving; as discussed from a biblical perspective and sound deductive reasoning as evident in positive results (Philippians 4:6).

# TABLE OF CONTENTS

# INTRODUCTION

When Marqwetta Johnson collapsed in her Tulsa, Oklahoma home, she had no idea that she was pregnant. Before she could be transported to the hospital and given the appropriate care, she was far too gone. She suffered a condition known as ectopic pregnancy, a condition that would have been easily treatable had it been discovered on time. But Marqwetta could not seek help. Being quite poor herself, and having seven children to take care of, she could hardly spare the funds to dedicate to seeking medical care. This is not surprising because Marqwetta was black.

Sad as it is, Marqwetta's story is actually not unique. Quite often (more often than necessary), we hear the stories of black women who die from pregnancy complications, sometimes from situations that could have been easily resolved. This scourge is spread across every stratum of the black demography. From the wealthy and powerful, such as Serena Williams, to poor women living in slums and poor neighborhoods, no one is spared. These women are all united by the unique tones of their skins and the knowledge of the fact that their medical system will, at some point, fail them, if it has not already done so. Their names dot the landscape – Shalon Irving, Courdeja West, Marqwetta Johnson, indictments against a system that is rigged against them and shows no signs of letting up now or in the future.

African American women contribute 43.5 percent of the total maternal mortality rate in the United States, according to the Center for Disease Control and Prevention. This simply means that African American mothers contribute three out of every five infant deaths in the country. Thus, even though infant and maternal mortality affects women from all backgrounds, the situation of African American women has become so severe, necessitating special attention.

The prospects are bleak, and if you are worried, you sure have good cause to be. This book seeks to explore the history and causes of this wide margin that exists between these two groups. This is done with the assumption, if not the hope, that an identification of the causes would also lead to the solutions. Hence, this book also contains some actionable steps that can be taken, both by the individual, the state, and every other stakeholder in the medical community. We would be dishonest to believe that we have anything short of an emergency on our hands. It thus behooves us to treat it as such.

## Chapter One

# UNDERSTANDING THE HISTORY OF THE HIGH INFANT AND MATERNAL MORTALITY RATES IN THE UNITED STATES

A terrible maternal and infant mortality rate is a legacy that has trailed the American society. This is to say that the deplorable state of black maternal and infant mortality rate is symptomatic of a pattern that exists in the larger American healthcare system. This is sad because as the American society is setting the pace in various other spheres, from academics to tech to even sports, one segment that is supposed to be the beacon of civilization still lags behind. What this depicts is that, sadly, American society has not made as much progress as it should from the days when crude implements were used to perform surgeries in the backrooms of houses.

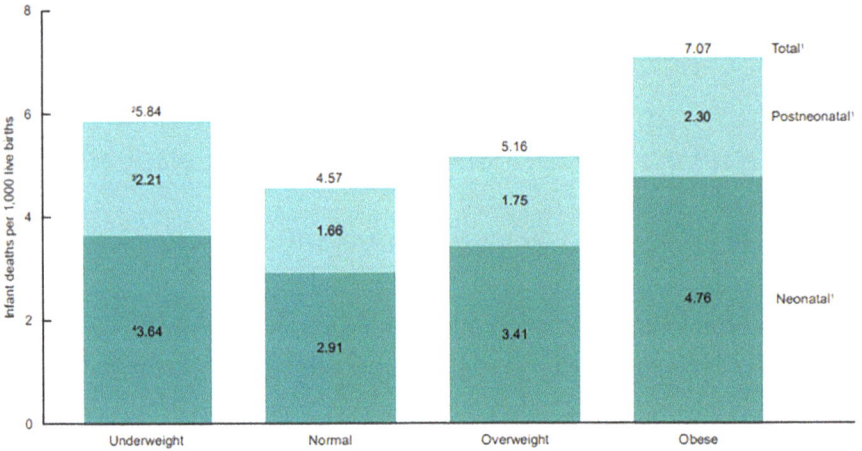

Figure 1: Infant mortality rates, by maternal pregnancy body mass index and infant age of death: United States, 2017 – 2018.

Source: https://www.cdc.gov/nchs//nvsr/nvsr69/NVSR-69-09-508.pdf

The United States of America holds the record of the highest infant mortality rate in the world. During the maternal period, mothers in the United States are thrice more likely to die than those in Canada. The maternal period is taken to be the time from pregnancy to one year after birth. Of course, consideration has to be given to the slight discrepancies in the recording metrics of countries all over the world. However, it remains undisputed that the maternal mortality rate in the United States is extremely high. The same is the case with infant mortality. For instance, infants in the United States have a more than a 76 percent mortality rate than others in developed nations, similar to the United States.

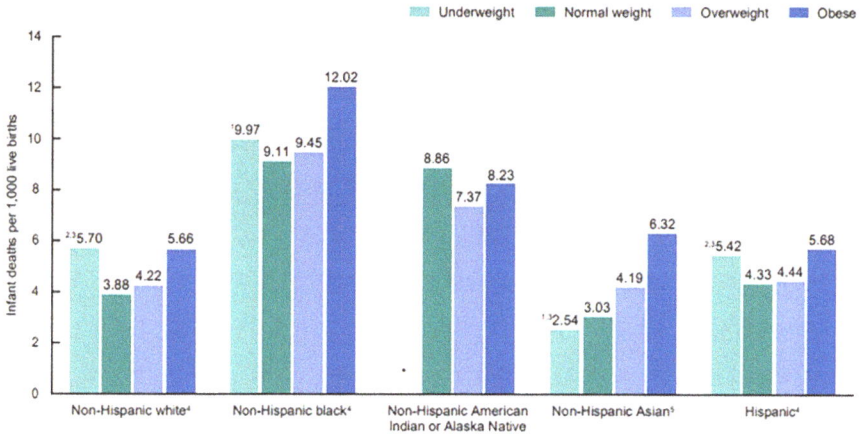

Figure 2: Infant Mortality rates by maternal pre-pregnancy body mass index and race and Hispanic origin: United States, 2018.

Source: https://www.cdc.gov/nchs/data/nvsr/nvsr69/NVSR-69-09-508.pdf

This general mortality crisis could perhaps explain, in part, the high mortality rate among African American mothers in the United States. It is true that maternal mortality rates in the United States experienced a sharp decline at the beginning of the 20th century. For instance, the infant death per 1000 babies was at 5.79, translating to 22,000 babies dying before their first birthday in 2017. This is an improvement from earlier years. In fact, the rate has gone 16 percent up than from 2005. However, the mortality rates are climbing back up, with the rates for African American women leading the pack. For instance, a report suggests that babies born to black women were more likely to die from complications resulting from preterm related issues than the case for non-Hispanic white women. The rate is thrice that for white women and holds true as recent as 2017. This is a trend that cuts across the different sublevels in the African American community. From the lowly stay-at-home spouse to the stupendously wealthy – such as the tennis star,

Serena Williams –the black mother is at greater risk of losing her life during childbirth as against their Caucasian or Hispanic counterparts.

Maternal deaths can also offer explanations for infant mortality as well. It is instructive to bear in mind that more than half of infant deaths occur before the first month of the child's existence elapses. These deaths are usually tied to preterm complications in a vast majority of cases. Preterm births severely plague African American women within the United States. It is on record that African American women have the highest number of preterm births. This also then provides the reason African Americans have the highest number of infant deaths compared to any other racial group.

## Tracing the History of the Disparity in Maternal and Child Mortality Rates for African American Women

Although much information does not exist or has been lost about maternal mortality rate before 1900, some conclusions can still be reached with existent data. Judging from independent research carried out by researchers such as John Billing, his conclusion, made from the 1880 census, was that there were more than 5 deaths per one thousand for births by black mothers, as opposed to 3 to one thousand for their white counterparts. In fact, maternal mortality was such an important feature that it was reported to be the cause of death for more than 25 percent of all reported deaths amongst black females. This is as opposed to just 14 percent for white females. Following from 1915 and upwards, comprehensive records about maternal and infant mortality rates were available. Records show that within that period, there were, on average, 11 deaths per thousand for black females.

Figure 3:

1987

**7.2**

American mothers died
per 100,000 live births.

2014

**18**

American mothers died
per 100,000 live births.

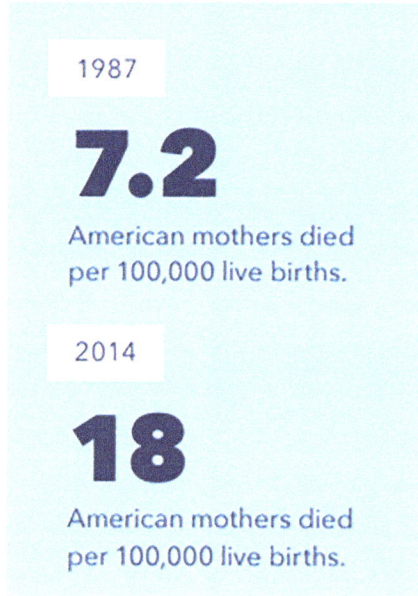

Source: https://www.plannedparenthood.org/uploads/filer_public/60/63/606313ba-556c-485b-bf3f-327cc2d50863/191017-maternal-mortality-fact-sheet-p02.pdf

It is impossible to deny the role race plays in the disparity in the discussion about the disparity in maternal and infant mortality rates in the United States. A look back at history will, perhaps, shed more light on why this is true. For instance, in 1662, Virginia legislators passed a law following a principle known as *partus sequitur ventrem*. This principle states that a child's status would follow its mother. This may seem innocuous, but is anything but. The principle was just a further perpetuation of chattel slavery.

It simply made chattel slavery an inheritable enterprise, giving slave owners the legal rights not only over the women themselves but also the offspring of these women. This is because, as owners of the slaves, they also owned whatever the slaves owned, including their offspring. One indicator of the nefarious intentions cloaking the legislation is the intent focus European exploration literature paid to the child-bearing abilities of African American women.

It would have been expected that at the end of the civil war, and with both the United States and England abolishing slavery, that things would get better. However, that was hardly the case. The ban on transatlantic slavery cut off the overseas supply of slaves for slave owners, especially in the antebellum South. However, these owners then began to rely on their fertile slave women to continue to produce offspring for them. This period, white physicians began to pay a lot of attention to the reproductive health of black women. Before this time, black women provided the help and necessary care needed when a slave was pregnant and during the delivery process.

However, the tides changed, and on the surface might be argued that this was for the best as these women got the best possible care during this period, but it was also a means through which these owners kept the slaves in line. Regardless of this measure, maternal and infant mortality continued to be high on the plantations. It was reported that in some cases, no less than 50 percent of infants born to slave women died within one year of birth. If the slave owners had not been fixated on just making rearing horses of these women, they might have realized that to reduce mortality rates, comprehensive care has to be given to the slaves.

This would have entailed a reduction of the workload, coupled with appropriate nutrition for these pregnant women. It would have been then that these women would have even stood the chance of reducing the maternal mortality rates. But, of course, it would have been economically unwise for these slave owners to expend funds to cater to these women. However, what this resulted in was the death of black slaves during childhood, leading to a loss eventually for the owners.

Apart from the treatment slave women faced at the hands of their slave owners, they also had a precarious relationship with the physicians. On the one hand, these physicians treated the women as nothing more than chattel, neither devoting the time or resources needed to improve their care. Even more so, these physicians often used black bodies as the site for many of their surgical adventures. Many of the groundbreaking techniques that have entered mainstream medicine have their origin from the bodies of black women.

These women had to endure countless experiments, some of them horrendous. For instance, James Marion Sims honed his technique used for the repair of the obstetrical fistula by practicing on the body or black women time and again. Furthermore, we perhaps would not have cesarean section surgeries like we do today if Francois Marie Prevost had not taken the liberties that he did with slave women.

Figure 4:

**Maternal Mortality Rate in the United States**
1900 - 1990

**NUMBER OF PREGNANCY-RELATED DEATHS PER 100,000 LIVE BIRTHS**

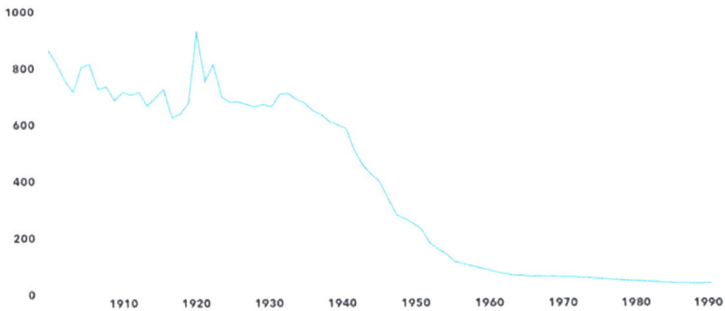

Source: https://www.plannedparenthood.org/uploads/filer_public/60/63/606313ba-556c-485b-bf3f-327cc2d50863/191017-maternal-mortality-fact-sheet-p02.pdf

It goes without saying that the American health system would forever be indebted to, and cannot hope to atone for, these acts carried out on black bodies. Although this cannot be directly linked to the high mortality rate in black communities, it can at least explain the skepticism with which black women view the American healthcare system. Decades of this trauma having lived with the black community; it is no surprise that women have a deep-rooted distrust for doctors generally. But even more so, it is apparent that doctors have yet to unlearn the levity with which they treat concerns of black women.

The vestiges of slavery still reverberate through the times, manifesting in various ways, in this instance, through the maternal mortality rate of black women. Even though since 1994, maternal and infant mortality rates across the world dropped by more than 50 percent, this cannot be said to be the case for the United States. For instance, between 2000 and 2013, the United States was the country with the second-highest mortality rate out of 31 countries polled.

It might be important to point out that there exist disparities between the infant and maternal mortality rates of African American women and African immigrant women in the United States. The infant and maternal mortality rates of the latter are lower. In fact, African immigrant women have almost the same maternal mortality ratio as non-Hispanic white women. On the surface, what this suggests is that African women, wherever they are found, have a strong disposition towards higher incidences of infant mortality. However, arriving as this conclusion would be a hasty enterprise, if not a wrong one entirely. This is because, upon examination, it will be seen that these immigrant women, at some point, begin to have the same infant and maternal death rates as African American women in the United States.

Over time, incidences of preterm births, as well as low birth weight, increase exponentially, suggesting that it is the American system, and not necessarily the disposition of these women that contributes to the high mortality rates. If anything, this goes to show how racial discrimination continues to affect African American women. Researchers have pinned these discrepancies as to the accumulation of years of weathering racial discrimination. This culminates in a weakened immune system and thus invariably affects pregnancy and childbirth.

*Chapter Two*

# EXAMINING THE CAUSES OF MATERNAL MORTALITY AMONG AFRICAN AMERICANS

## 1. Racism

If racism appears to be a recurring decimal in this discourse, it is only because of how important a role it plays. The mere fact that color is the dividing line between different ethnic groups when it comes to maternal mortality rate lends credence to this assertion. However, even beyond speculations, there is irrefutable proof to show that racism is the most significant determinant of the differences in maternal mortality rates.

African Americans have endured decades of racism in the United States. It is a reality that is intricately tied to the idea and identity of the black person in the United States. Racism itself has compromised various structures, rigging the system to the disfavor of blacks. This is to say that the effects of racism are pervasive, and scarcely any sector escapes its taint. From the judicial system – where a disproportionate number of black people fill the prisons, to the educational structures and facilities available to the black person, and even in entertainment. Racism experienced in the healthcare system is just one example of this system that has existed for eons.

This system where the public structures are used to perpetuate racial inequality is known as structural racism. This is traceable to the fact that the structures are predominantly white-owned and is weighted against people of color. What this means is that African American mothers receive a lower quality of care than their white counterparts. Structural racism is also seen in the quick dismissal of complaints of African American women, sometimes even by the healthcare providers and social service personnel tasked with providing them with care. Racism also predisposes African American women to a wide range of pregnancy-related problems such as preeclampsia, eclampsia, and embolisms (all of these will be discussed at length subsequently.)

The effects of racism on the emotional and physical health of African American women also get transferred to their offspring. Medical problems that are peculiar to infants such as Sudden Infant Death Syndrome (SIDS), Sudden Unexpected Infant Death (SUD) is high among women of color, a testament to the effects of structural racism. It is true that the United States has one of the highest rates of the use of C-section in deliveries (This is important because cesarean births come with higher complications and risks that are oftentimes absent, or at least mitigated, in the case of vaginal births.) However, even in this regard, black women are offered the option of, and sometimes forced to accept, c-section more than non-Hispanic white women and women from non-minority races. For instance, in 2017, the rate of c-section births between black women and Caucasians was 36 percent to 30 percent. Little wonder then that the rate of SIDs/SUD deaths was almost twice the rate for non-Hispanic black women.

**Figure 5: Causes of Infant Mortality**

**Infant deaths and mortality rates for the top 5 leading causes of death for African Americans, 2017 (Rates per 100,000 live births)**

| Cause of Death (By rank) | # African American Deaths | African American Death Rate | #Non-Hispanic White Deaths | Non-Hispanic White Death Rate | African American / Non-Hispanic White Ratio |
|---|---|---|---|---|---|
| (1) Low-Birth weight | 1,354 | 241.5 | 1,260 | 63.2 | 3.8 |
| (2) Congenital Malformations | 822 | 146.6 | 2,138 | 107.3 | 1.4 |
| (3) Maternal Complications | 467 | 83.3 | 470 | 23.6 | 3.5 |
| (4) Accidents (unintentional injuries) | 397 | 70.8 | 619 | 31.1 | 2.3 |
| (5) Sudden infant death syndrome (SIDS) | 391 | 69.7 | 688 | 34.5 | 2.0 |

## 2. Under investing in family support and programs

Over the years, there have been ongoing concerns that the government pays little or no attention to issues regarding maternal and infant health. In fact, the programs that even exist, such as Medicaid, Temporary Assistance for Needy Families (TANF), have had their funds reduced or out rightly cut out. Viewed from a skeptic lens, this may seem to be a deliberate act by the powers that be to perpetuate the subjugation of blacks. In any case, there is no doubt that this is a symptom of, if not a fruit of, structural racism.

The effects of this lack of attention paid to family support are most felt by black families who rely on this support. Black women who used to depend on subsidy from the government during their period of pregnancy suddenly find themselves without any recourse. It then comes as no surprise that a sudden rise in maternal and infant deaths in the black community is the outcome.

## 3. Lack of prenatal care

The essence of prenatal care is to provide assistance for pregnant mothers through the pregnancy process and ensure that safe delivery is achieved. Healthcare experts engage in activities which include parent education, counseling on healthy practices and behaviors etc. to make sure that pregnant women are quite aware of the dangers they put themselves in when they fail to take the necessary actions to protect themselves and their babies.

In fact, no research, but common sense, is required to make the argument those women who receive prenatal care from health experts experience better health outcomes. Viewed in this light, another factor that contributes to the high infant and maternal mortality rates amongst the black community can be identified. Research shows that more black women lack access to prenatal care than non-Hispanic black women.

This lack of access can be explained on the basis of racism and other structural handicaps that black people face. For instance, there is a lack of sensitization and awareness about the potential risks associated with rejecting prenatal care in many black communities. Families who live in the ghettos are the worst hit because of the deep distrust that exists between health establishments and these neighborhoods. What this means is that black mothers do not access prenatal care even when they can afford to. The outcome then is seen in the differences in the deaths experienced in the first trimester between black and non-Hispanic white women.

What this also indicates is that there can be a quick reversal of this status. If black communities can commit to accessing prenatal care, when necessary, the rate of maternal and infant deaths within the black community will be drastically reduced.

## Neglect of key Physical health factors

There are a lot of physical health factors that affect birth outcomes. These factors incorporate physical behaviors that can influence pregnancy outcomes regardless of the race of the person involved. The factors that are most touted as influencing maternal and infant mortality are drug abuse, smoking, and obesity. It is important to note that none of these factors can singly account for the high maternal and infant mortality rate in the black community. However, the fact that those three exists in abundance in the community can lend credence to the assertion that they affect maternal and infant mortality. An examination of each of these factors singly is essential to get the full picture.

**Figure 6: Percentage of mothers who smoked during pregnancy, 2017**

| Non-Hispanic Black | Non-Hispanic White | Non-Hispanic Black / Non-Hispanic White Ratio |
|:---:|:---:|:---:|
| 5.6 | 10.1 | 0.6 |

Source: CDC 2019. Births: Final Data for 2017 National Vital Statistics Reports. Table13. https://www.cdc.gov/nchs/data/nvsr/nvsr67/nvsr67_08-508.pdf

Smoking and drug abuse have been linked to risk situations such as low-birth-weight, preterm delivery, and infant death syndrome. Yet, there is a high rate of drug use reported with pregnant black women. Again, families that live in ghettos and slums are at higher risks. Even more so, studies show that black women were less likely to report smoking habits and the problems that come with it than non-Hispanic white women. This, of course, means that diagnosis and identification of health complications from smoking and drug abuse are not afforded these women. Thus, even apart from the fact that these women were more likely to abuse drugs and alcohol, they were still less likely to get the help required to counteract the effects of these habits.

Furthermore, obesity is a risk factor that predicts such conditions, such as preeclampsia. Research has also shown that there is a high tolerance for, and rate of, obesity in the black community. Of course, the expectation will be that this risk factor will predispose black women to higher maternal and infant deaths, but there is no consensus on that yet. There is no data that directly links the high level of obesity in the black community with fatal maternal and infant deaths.

In fact, research shows that African women of normal weight experienced greater risks of death during pregnancy than obese African American women. It might be important to point out that the lack of conclusive evidence is no indication at all. What is certain is that obesity and such risky behaviors such as drug and alcohol abuse pose threats to pregnant mothers and should be strongly discouraged within the black community.

## 4. The structure of the American healthcare system

It does bear repeating that the structure of the health system unfairly targets people of color, women especially. However, apart from the healthcare sector, almost every other sector contributes to the high maternal and infant mortality rate. For instance, it is the truth that people of color are concentrated in the poorest neighborhoods. These communities also lack quality health facilities and programs.

Additionally, these areas have the most exposure to toxins and environmental hazards, lack favorable laws and policies, and generally have policies that are not favorable to pregnant women, regardless of their race. Thus, it happens that the fact that African American women are found concentrated in these areas, the reflection is in the number of mortality rates both for mothers and children.

Furthermore, the intersection of racism with other forms of bias also results in unfavorable outcomes for women of color. It is true that external factors such as sexual orientation, income level, education, disability can affect maternal mortality rates, albeit indirectly. In this particular case, there is the intersection of racism and sexism. Hence, it appears that there are two strikes against women of color already. The twin forces of racism and sexism result in the lack of attention paid to black and Asian women in healthcare settings. This dismissal of the complaints of women leads to feelings of invisibility and inferiority.

Thus, when such women are hesitant about approaching hospitals when they experience complications associated with a pregnancy, they can hardly be blamed. This ingrained system of silence and dismissal has resulted in women being afraid, or at least wary of speaking up in situations where they experience shabby healthcare services from healthcare practitioners.

## 5. Mental Health Factors

Undoubtedly, the level of stress a pregnant woman experiences can impact pregnancy outcomes. Stress and other mental health-related issues can increase the risk of abortions and maternal deaths during pregnancy. Generally, there does not appear to be any difference between the stress level of African women and non-Hispanic white women. However, this could easily be explained by the fact that a great proportion of these women may not have access to facilities that can enable them to diagnose and identify mental health issues or even take a step further to request treatment.

Women of color are also often unaware of the signs of mental health challenges during and after pregnancy. Additionally, women of color are less likely to report mental health challenges than non-Hispanic white women. This can be linked to the severe distrust that exists between the medical establishments and people of color generally. A peculiar reason that could explain why women of color fail to get health for mental health-related issues during pregnancy is the insufficiency of the body of knowledge available on the subject.

The information available about how to identify and properly diagnose these issues fails to take into cognizance the peculiarities of black folks. Women of color experience stressors on several levels. This includes, but is not limited, to issues relating to racism, sexism, and other forms of gender-based discrimination, especially in the workplace. Thus, before any comprehensive action can be taken to eliminate mental health-related issues peculiar to black women, a holistic view of the subject should be entertained.

## 6. Underlying Diseases

One of the highest causes of maternal and infant mortality deaths generally is underlying sicknesses. Women who present with illnesses at the start of their pregnancies often find it difficult to carry their babies to term in a vast majority of cases. However, black women are more likely to present with underlying illnesses than their non-Hispanic counterparts. Some of the diseases that affect pregnant women include preeclampsia, hypertension, and eclampsia. Preeclampsia and eclampsia are quite common among pregnant women, at least more common than should be the case.

In fact, the global prevalence of preeclampsia is at 5 percent. They can occur even more than six weeks after delivery, although they are common within the first six weeks and with women who were having their first babies. Also, risk factors include obesity, preexisting hypertension, and diabetes. Given that these risk factors, particularly obesity, are high within the black community, it is no surprise then that infant death, fallout of these diseases, is then high in the black community.

Another medical condition that impacts maternal and infant mortality rate is obstetric hemorrhage. Hemorrhage can occur pre/postpartum. Excessive bleeding can occur because of abortion/early baby loss, problems with the placenta, as well as childbirth problems. In some cases, placenta eruptions prior to the birth of the baby can result in hemorrhage also. In the same vein, postpartum hemorrhage is also a leading cause of maternal and infant mortality globally. Just like the discussion above, the risk factors for hemorrhage include obesity, late pregnancy, and even previous cesarean births. These factors again are common with women of color, putting them at risk of hemorrhage and, thus, maternal and infant mortality.

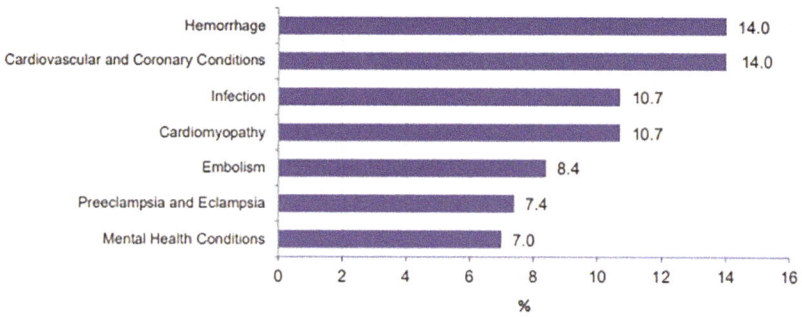

**Figure 7: Leading Underlying Causes of Pregnancy-Related Deaths**

`Source:https://reviewtoaction.org/sites/default/files/national-portal-material/
Report%20from%20Nine%20MMRCs%20final_0.pdf

## Chapter Three

# MEANS OF REDUCING INFANT MORTALITY RATES IN THE AFRICAN AMERICAN COMMUNITY

Even though the numbers are bleak at this moment, all hope is not lost. There are several steps that could be taken to bring down the high mortality rate in the black community. However, it will be no mean fit. It would require concerted efforts from the government and individuals alike. It is only in a collaborative environment that these issues can be addressed adequately, to the point of witnessing a turnaround, especially in terms of seeing a downturn of numbers.

Considering that these problems have a definitive racial tint to them, it would necessarily imply that policy decisions have to be taken. Policymakers, nay everyone in a position of government, has to factor in marginalized communities in their decision-making process. This would, of course, mean that these individuals would have to prioritize black people. Even within that demographic, certain subsets would need to be paid attention to. Thus, black people living in low-income communities who are often the worst hit in the medical crisis have to be prioritized.

The solutions, as discussed here, are divided into two parts: direct and non-direct solution mechanisms. Direct means refer to the actions which engage the health sector directly. Solutions here refer to the actions that have direct consequences for the people themselves. Indirect solution mechanisms refer to suggested solutions which do not directly affect black women and infants. These include policy actions, including the treatment of pregnant women in jails, the allocation for health facilities in poor black neighborhoods, as well as research into issues peculiar to black women and infants. Altogether these two factions provide a comprehensive framework that could be used to tackle infant and maternal mortality rates in the black community.

## Direct Plans For The Elimination/Reduction Of Maternal And Infant Mortality Rates In The Black Community

### 1. Pay attention to preterm births in black women

A baby is said to be preterm if it is born less than 37 weeks into the pregnancy. Preterm birth is one major cause of infant deaths, with numbers being as high as 17 percent in 2017. Apart from preterm birth being a direct cause of death, it can also be an indirect cause of infant death. For instance, a preterm baby is susceptible to diseases such as respiratory diseases and bacterial infections because of their compromised immune systems. Even more so, preterm births account for the gaping gap in the difference between the infant mortality rates between African American women and non-Hispanic black women.

All the causes of preterm birth are indeed unknown. In fact, at the time of writing this, the CDC is fervently carrying out research to determine the causes of preterm births. However, certain actions can be taken to diagnose and prevent it. For instance, certain behaviors such as smoking, unfavorable work conditions as well as drug abuse can be risk factors. More so, certain health conditions, including diabetes, high blood pressure, and infections, can increase the chances of preterm births in certain women.

Health experts should then be mindful of finding out if pregnant women had any of these underlying conditions. As already pointed out earlier, the long history of distrust between health institutions and the black community means that it would be near impossible to obtain accurate data through self-reportage. Hence, health officials ought to look for avenues to build trust with these women, while also looking for ingenious ways to gather accurate data about these conditions from the women concerned.

Apart from conducting screening and tests, these health officials can also measure the cervix as a way to prevent preterm births. There is a growing body of research that points to the fact that measuring a woman's cervix can be a means to detect those at high risk. It is important to bear in mind that cervix shortening is one of the first signs of labor. This also means that making use of a sonogram to detect early shortening of the cervix can be a means to predict and prevent preterm births. The administering of progesterone has also been credited with helping combat preterm risks. Progesterone is a hormone that is crucial for pregnancy, being responsible for reducing contractions. It should, of course, be mentioned that this remedy might not be good for all women. For example, it would typically not work for women who have had multiple births.

On the part of policymakers, they have the responsibility of making policies that will increase access to these screening services. The steps to achieving this include carrying out vigorous outreach and sensitization programs, allocation of more funds, and also provision of the necessary assistance for the treatment of these diseases when they arise. Also, they have to further create an enabling environment for black women to feel safe enough to volunteer these pieces of information when required to.

| CARDIOVASCULAR AND CORONARY CONDITIONS | HEMORRHAGE |
|---|---|
| Improve training | Improve training |
| Adopt maternal levels of care/Ensure appropriate level of care determination | Adopt maternal levels of care/Ensure appropriate level of care determination |
| Improve procedures related to communication and coordination between providers | Improve procedures related to communication and coordination between providers |
| Improve standards regarding assessment, diagnosis, and treatment decisions | Improve standards regarding assessment, diagnosis, and treatment decisions |
| Improve policies related to patient management, communication and coordination between providers, and language translation | Improve policies related to patient management, communication and coordination between providers, and language translation |
| Improve access to care | Improve patient/provider communication |
| Improve policies regarding prevention initiatives | Enforce policies/procedures |
| | Mandate autopsies |

Figure 8: Recommended Steps to Eliminate Cardiovascular problems and hemorrhage.

## 2. Increase access to midwives

It is no secret that a vast majority of black moms do not get the best of care during their prenatal days. The cause of this, amongst, include poverty. A lot of black mothers cannot afford to pay a midwife to see them through the process of childbirth. Thus, if Medicaid covers the prenatal services offered by midwives and doulas, better positive outcomes may be guaranteed.

Specifically, research has found that doulas provide more visible care for black women who are in a low-income neighborhood or disadvantaged in any other way. Even more so, one-on-one care from doulas has been known to produce the best outcomes. This is because this kind of personal care fosters intimacy and trust between both parties. The result of this is greater positive birth outcomes for patients, who, in this case, will be black women. In the same vein, midwives have been known to increase the odds of a favorable birth for mothers generally. The benefits that result from midwifery include an overall reduction in preterm births, as well as a lower neonatal loss.

States do not typically cover doulas in their medical funding programs. Furthermore, private health insurance fails to consider this too. Statistically, less than 1 percent of American states provide coverage for doula services. At the time of writing this, only two states, Minnesota and Oregon, provide support for doula services in their Medicaid options. On the other hand, all states incorporate support for Medicaid services in their programs. However, the scope of the financial support provided depends on several factors, including the qualifications of the midwife concerned.

Historically, African American women dominated the midwifery practice. However, all these changed when stricter measures were implemented, which were intended to make it harder for women of color to scale through. Thus, in instituting policies to include the access to midwives for black pregnant mothers, education of black midwives needs to be prioritized.

## 3. Implement the use of infant screening

There are conditions that may lie undetected for a long time in the infant, except adequate tests are carried out. These inherent conditions may have the effect of shortening the lifespan of the newborn if not detected and treated on time. In fact, an infant suffering any of such conditions may appear fine and then die a few days afterward from unknown causes. This is the reality for black babies many times too often.

Thus, these screenings must be done as soon as possible. The process is uncomplicated. It usually involves drawing blood from the baby and then carrying out tests to screen for these conditions. The conditions tested for are usually between 40 and above. Certain factors such as the family history of the child, the state of the child's mother, etc. can influence the number of tests to be carried out.

## 4. Tackling racism and implicit bias

As much as it is the desire of every black person to see racism in all forms eradicated totally, the truth is that it may be slow in coming. Total elimination of racism may appear to be a tall order because of several reasons, including the fact that the institutions that reinforce racism have been in existence for centuries and may not be dismantled easily. Hence, one has to settle for a systemic and continuous tackling of racism. One area that this fight needs to be fought valiantly is the medical sector.

The truth is that disparities in the attention given to non-Hispanic white women, and black women are sometimes quite subtle and indecipherable. They can manifest in such forms as dismissing concerns raised by women of color, giving different treatment recommendations, or even under treating pain in some cases. This can be addressed by teaching medical officers to become aware of how implicit bias may color their relations with black patients. They will need to become more culturally sensitive, as well as understand that (as a white person), they may never understand the full range of the difficulties faced by a black woman.

For policymakers, proper funding needs to be provided to ensure the education of every person that comes in contact with pregnant black women are culturally sensitive. Models can also be created where medical personnel take some time to work in underdeveloped communities in order to get firsthand knowledge of the black experience. Certain misconceptions pervade the medical space about the physiological markup of black people. For instance, one of such is the assumption that black people are able to endure pain more, an attitude which leads to the dismissal of complaints by black people. However, when these people work within black communities, they will be disabused of these notions.

The truth is that even though a wholesome body of research chronicles racial disparities in the medical community, much more needs to be done. Further research needs to be carried into healthcare settings with the aim of identifying ways of tackling these racial inequalities. Policymakers need to set aside funds to enable these researches to be carried out. It is even more important to make sure that there is adequate representation in the individuals carrying out the research. These individuals, apart from having the requisite credentials, will also be armed with lived experiences that will be essential to identifying and stamping out racism.

## 5. Reduce the use of C-sections

A C-section (also known as a Caesarean birth) is a process where the fetus is cut from the mother's womb through surgical means. It is an alternative for birthing naturally where it is impossible, or medically inadvisable, for the mother to go through vaginal birth. Usually, C-sections carry more risks both for the mother and the fetus than vaginal births. It is for this reason that the rate of maternal and infant mortality is higher from cases of C-sections than vaginal births. The complications that could arise from C-sections include injury to the fetus, postpartum hemorrhage, etc.

These risks can be some grave that they could even affect future pregnancies. The United States has one of the highest rates of C-section births all over the world. It is also one of the most frequent surgeries conducted, with states such as Florida, Mississippi having up to 37 percent of all births conducted through C-sections. To put things in a better perspective: 1 out of every 3 children given birth to in the United States was through C-sections. More so, black women are more likely to have their babies through C-sections, as opposed to other racial categories.

In light of the many complications associated with C-sections, it goes without saying then that reducing the rate of the use of C-sections will reduce these risks. This is even as the World Health Organization has stipulated that a C-section rate above 10 percent of the population is inimical to the elimination of infant and maternal mortality rates.

## 6. Increase in health literacy and childbirth education

Indeed, one of the leading causes of the high infant and maternal mortality rates in the black community is ignorance. Thus, concerted efforts should be made to provide an education of, and re-education of pregnant black women. The body of knowledge that should be provided these women should be comprehensive, encompassing the various risk areas associated with childbirth, especially within the black community. The effect of these efforts will culminate in these women acquiring the skills that will help them identify and understand health information regarding their peculiar situations.

The government and other stakeholders in the sector need to provide funding for health literacy education. In this regard, programs led by people of color should be prioritized. This is because grassroots mobilization and sensitization is always necessary for reaching disadvantaged communities. An example of an outfit spearheading the sensitization campaign is the Ancient Song Doula Services. They teach maternal health-related topic such as health and legal rights, identification of health complications, and steps to seeking a remedy. Commendable as it is a fantastic job they are doing, there is the need for more organizations such as theirs to spring up.

## 7. Make a conscious effort to advocate for yourself during medical appointments.

Whether you have a doula or not, it is always a promising idea to be vocal about your needs and concerns during your medical appointments. It is sad that this is the reality, but the odds are that many doctors could potentially dismiss your concerns and ignore your symptoms, even when you know deep down that they are serious.

Again, it is a grim reality, but to protect both your own health and the health of your baby, make a point of standing up for yourself during your medical appointments. If your doctor seems dismissive, repeat your concerns: For example, "I know that you are not concerned about this symptom, but I truly believe that it's serious. Could you please run some more tests, or refer me to a specialist for a second opinion?" The doctor may get defensive or angry with you, but know that it is well within your rights to speak up for yourself when you think that you are being treated unfairly.

You must understand that if Serena Williams had not insisted about getting help concerning her symptoms, her fears would have been waved away. She would have lost her baby, and even maybe her life in the process. You must be quite firm about demanding for attention to be given to your demands. You may even go as far as going up the chain of command if your attending physician fails to acknowledge your concerns.

If you feel nervous about doing this alone, perhaps bring your partner, a family member, a close friend, or even your doula with you to your appointments so that they can chime in if they notice that you are being treated unfairly. Again, it is wrong that you even need to take these extremes measures in the first place, but being your own advocate can help mitigate the discrimination you may face.

## 8. Providing adequate mental health services

The mental health of pregnant women is often overlooked when the discourse is on the ways to prevent maternal and infant deaths. Even when the issue makes a rare appearance, it is not given adequate attention; an issue of such nature ought to be given. This apathy can be said to be uniform throughout the entire healthcare industry, for is it not only recently that some attention began to be paid to postpartum depression, even though it has been the leading medical health issue affecting pregnant women in the United States for several decades?

This attitude is, however, exacerbated in the case of African American women. The complaints of these women are dismissed and chalked up to baby blues and baby anxiety. Little wonder a report carried out in New Jersey from July 2004 to October 2007 showed that black women were almost twice less likely to report cases of postpartum depression or seek treatment for it. The study also showed that even in the instances where these women sought help, the health officials did not bother carrying out follow-up care to ensure that the women turned out fine.

A lot of women experience trauma for the first-time during pregnancy. Several reports have found that no less than 40 percent of women having babies for the first time had never experienced any sort of trauma prior to that time. This trauma can be compounded if some complications are experienced during the pregnancy or birth, or if the baby has complications after birth. Another aspect of trauma that needs to be handled is those related to sexual assault. Sexual assault which results in pregnancy can come with specific forms of trauma. For instance, women who have experienced sexual assault find it difficult to accept gynecological exams.

Also, they may find it difficult to have discussions about their sexual history and thus fail to obtain the help they need. An appreciable number of pregnancies reported by black women result from sexual assault. In fact, according to a report by the CDC in 2011, up to 22 percent of black women reported that they had been raped in their lifetimes. A further 41 percent reported that although they had never been raped, they had experienced sexual harassment and assault of varying degrees and nature. If these numbers appear high, consider the fact that a lot of women do not report cases of sexual assault. Thus, there is no doubt that the numbers are quite higher than they are.

Health officials ought to take into consideration these specific instances of trauma while offering help to patients. This is through a phenomenon known as trauma-informed care. Trauma-informed care is a comprehensive healthcare pattern that takes into consideration the history of trauma experienced by the patient. Thus, it may entail requesting for permission before touching the patient, explaining every step thoroughly to the patient, as well as asking for a trusted companion to be around during the examination process. It is important that the patient's hesitations and complaints be listened to.

| RECOMMENDATION | IMPACT LEVEL (%) | |
| --- | --- | --- |
| | SMALL TO MEDIUM | LARGE TO GIANT |
| Improve training | 72.7 | 27.3 |
| Enforce policies and procedures | 40.0 | 60.0 |
| Adopt maternal levels of care/Ensure appropriate level of care determination | 0.0 | 100.0 |
| Improve access to care | 50.0 | 50.0 |
| Improve patient/provider communication | -- | -- |
| Improve patient management for mental health conditions | 80.0 | 20.0 |
| Improve procedures related to communication and coordination between providers | 55.0 | 45.0 |
| Improve standards regarding assessment, diagnosis, and treatment decisions | 69.2 | 30.8 |
| Improve policies related to patient management, communication and coordination between providers, and language translation | 42.9 | 57.1 |
| Improve policies regarding prevention initiatives, including screening procedures and substance use prevention or treatment programs | 0.0 | 100.0 |

Figure 9: Potential Level of Impact of Recommendations

Source:https://reviewtoaction.org/sites/default/files/national-portal-material/Report%20from%20Nine%20MMRCs%20final_0.pdf

## Indirect means of reducing maternal and infant mortality rates

In this section, the discussion will focus on strategies that may not be directly focused on the mother and child. The discussion will encompass other segments such as the workplace, the criminal justice system, etc. The indirect actions that could potentially reduce infant and maternal mortality rates in black communities in the United States. These strategies include:

## 1. Improve workplace conditions

The workplace conditions of pregnant women and new mothers can have an impact on the health of their infants. Workplace conditions and policies that take cognizance of the unique situations of these women often lead to more favorable outcomes and reduce the instances of maternal and infant deaths. The reverse is usually the case when the conditions are otherwise. Unfortunately, the odds are stacked against women of color in this regard. Black women are more likely to work in low-income jobs. This invariably means that they get to work unfavorable hours without receiving benefits such as a great insurance plan, etc.

The Pregnancy Discrimination Act already exists, but its provisions are hardly enough, especially relating to the specific situations of African American women. Thus, more needs to be done. This could be in the form of creating a uniform national paid family and medical leave. This would make it possible for these women to take the time needed to recuperate after childbirth and also care for their babies without having to worry about exhausting their resources.

More so, affordable (if not free health care) should be made available to these women. In developing these policies, it is important that strategies to eliminate poverty should also be considered. This is because of the substantial proportion of black women who resort to these low-paying jobs because of the lack of options. This, coupled with institutional racism that makes it harder, if not impossible, for women of color to find meaningful employment, means that improving workplace conditions will only do so much if the root cause is not addressed.

## 2. Improve awareness of safe sleep behaviors

This is a general suggestion that could work both for black women and non-Hispanic white women alike. Close to 4,000 infant deaths are attributed to sleep-related causes each year. This is a problem associated not just with the new mothers of these infants, but also every other primary caregiver, or anyone who sleeps with an infant in close proximity. Sleep-related causes of death include, but are not limited to, smothering, asphyxiation (where the infant shares sleeping space with someone else), as well as babies falling off from their beds or cradle (when sleeping alone). It is important to improve awareness of safe sleep behaviors.

For these campaigns to work, they have to be informative and educational. They have to identify these problems exactly, and then address them, elaborating on the correct measures to take to eliminate sleep-related deaths. Furthermore, to increase the effectiveness of such campaigns, they have to be targeted at a specific group. As already stated, the groups targeted should include the mothers of these infants, caregivers, such as grandparents and nannies, etc. Specificity would thus mean that the medium to be used in each case would be appropriate for the targeted audience. For example, it would hardly make sense for adverts targeted at grandparents to be run on YouTube or the likes. Furthermore, if the target is towards ethnic groups with a high percentage of infant sleep-related deaths, then the peculiarities of said group should be incorporated into the sent messages.

## 3. Support for Breastfeeding

As remote as the possibility is, supporting breastfeeding can help reduce infant and maternal mortality rates within the black community. Support for breastfeeding is a wonderful tactic, but more so, support for workplace breastfeeding is quite essential. New mothers find it increasingly difficult to breastfeed their babies in hostile work environments. In fact, new mothers find it difficult to continue with their breastfeeding plans once they resume work. This can thus translate to increased anxiety and stress levels, which can invariably affect the general health conditions of the new mother and infant.

It is important to support and encourage breastfeeding because of the benefits it has both for the mother and the new child. Breastfeeding helps build the immune system of the newborn, providing essential nutrients that may be unavailable through any other means. It further helps in the elimination of infant diseases such as respiratory infections, gastrointestinal infections, SIDs, etc.

Special attention needs to be paid to black women. This is because they are the demography to return the earliest to work. Also, the fact that black women are mostly overrepresented in low-wage jobs also means that they often do not get enough leave to breastfeed their babies. These disparities in breastfeeding trends need to be addressed by policymakers. Incentives should be put in place to encourage robust workplace breastfeeding policies.

Finally, on this point, it is also important for the issue of workplace pregnancy discrimination to be addressed. The same way maternal and infant mortality rates are higher for African American women is the same way workplace pregnancy discrimination is higher for them too. There is hardly then any alternative explanation for why black women filed workplace discrimination lawsuits on a scale twice higher than the average for non-Hispanic white women in 2015.

The allegations of discrimination ranged from arbitrary firings, inadequate parental leave period, denial of promotions and raises, etc. In some cases, these discriminatory policies may feature harsh working conditions for pregnant women, which then results in health complications both for the mother and infant. In this category, black women are often overrepresented. Due to stereotypes that exaggerate the tolerance of black people to pain as well as physical strengths and fitness, employers are often unwilling to recognize how harsh working environments may affect black women.

## 4. Revamp the Criminal Justice System

Every available statistic shows that people of color are overrepresented in the criminal justice system. More than 60 percent of incarcerated inmates are blacks. The same can be same for black women in prisons. The result from this is that African American children are twice more likely to have one parent or guardian in prison than a non-Hispanic white child. The sad reality is that most of these women, who are mothers, are often locked up for minor offenses. Furthermore, a large number of these women are survivors of violence themselves, making them vulnerable in the criminal justice system. It is for this reason that there is a high likelihood of substance abuse by inmates and survivors from prison than otherwise.

In and of itself, incarcerating (pregnant) women comes with negative consequences for the health and psyche of these women. This is further exacerbated when considered against the fact that certain inhumane treatments are meted out to these women while in prison. For instance, one practice that has had a negative impact on incarcerated women but is still practiced nonetheless is shackling. Shackling is no longer practiced in federal prisons, having been outlawed in 2008. However, some state and private-owned prisons still make use of shackling as a compliance mechanism.

The Immigration and Customs Enforcement (ICE) Detention makes use of this as well. Shackling is an inhumane practice, which is reminiscent of the slavery era. It dehumanizes persons and results in both physical and mental trauma for the person shackled. For women specifically, shackling can lead to complications related to delayed vaginal examination, resulting in maternal deaths. The government and other policy stakeholders need to take a decisive step to end shackling. Over the years, a lot of human rights groups have campaigned for the elimination of shackling, but the rate of development of regulations in this sector has been rather slow and sluggish.

Furthermore, strict regulations should be adopted by ICE concerning the treatment of incarcerated women. Generally, the practice of targeting women of color specifically should also be addressed. In recent times, it appears as though the discriminatory policies implemented by ICE against black women increased almost ten-fold. A comprehensive criminal justice reform will incorporate plans not only to ban the shackling of incarcerated women but also plans to eliminate the unfair targeting of women of color.

Additionally, quality healthcare services should be provided for incarcerated pregnant women. This should be the prerogative of stakeholders both in the private and public sectors. Only a few states provide for mandatory prenatal and postnatal care for incarcerated pregnant women. Furthermore, it is also important that prenatal nutrition be made non-negotiable. This is all in a bid to reduce the level of stress already experienced by these women as a result of their incarceration. People living with HIV/AIDS should also be paid keen attention to during this period. STIs and other infections can compromise the immune system of pregnant women, leading to the miscarriage of fetuses in some severe cases. Officials of these prisons should uphold the highest level of care for these women, even going as far as providing enough bonding time between incarcerated mothers and their infants after delivery.

*Chapter Four*

# EFFORTS AT ELIMINATING HIGH INFANT AND MATERNAL MORTALITY RATES IN BLACK COMMUNITIES

Even though our institutions and systems contribute, in part, to the high infant and maternal mortality rates in black communities, some sectors within the government are at the forefront of the fight for the elimination of these scary figures. It is important to point this out if only to acknowledge what they are doing. More so, it could stand as a signpost for African American women, showing them where they can obtain help when they need same.

## 1. Improved data collection

It is worthy of note that the Centre for Disease Control (CDC) had begun in 1986, to conduct surveillance on pregnancy-related deaths. The efforts included the development of a national tracking database, to keep an eye on the number of women dying from causes related to pregnancies. These efforts were so effective that several states in the United States adopted that same model and established their own tracking systems. These models are important because they help in providing the data and research necessary for the formulation of better policies for tackling this menace.

It is as a response to the disturbing data gathered from these tracking systems that the U.S Department of Health and Human Services proceeded with the first national strategy to address infant mortality in 2012. This national strategy then led to the formation of the Infant Mortality Collaborative Improvement and Innovation Network (COIIN). This agency is tasked with identifying and highlighting efforts at infant mortality reduction at local levels.

## 2. Efforts of some states

It is worthy of note that some states are focused in their fight against infant and maternal mortality rates in the United States. For instance, states like North Carolina and California have developed robust research facilities to identify and promote better outcomes for mothers and infants. Also, several advocates are carrying out efforts to raise awareness about the pitiable state of maternal and infant mortality rates, generally in the United States. On the other hand, there are also other advocacy groups focused on raising awareness for the plight of black mothers in the United States. Groups like National Birth Equity Collaborative are at the forefront of the fight to identify and eradicate factors that lead to the death of black mothers and infants in the country.

Regardless of this, there is still the need to do more. More research must be carried out in this area to make available accurate data that will aid the fight against maternal and infant mortality. At present, some knowledge gaps exist, which research alone will be able to fill. For instance, there is an urgent need for information that traces the correlation between race, economic status, geography with death rates. More so, the impact of racism, both on a large scale and in the minuscule versions it may be exhibited, on infant and maternal deaths. Accurate data should also be available to document the health status of mothers before, after, and during childbirth, to pinpoint exactly where the factors that increase maternal deaths creep in through.

## 3. Innovative Strategies by some states

Some states are introducing innovative plans that aim to address the problems of high maternal and infant deaths in the black community. Some of these efforts involve the use of technology. One of such introductions is the use of telehealth services. Offering telehealth services is one of the best ways to incorporate technology in the fight against maternal and infant deaths. It involves the use of tools such as video conferencing for the diagnosis and treatment of high-risk women.

This move automatically eliminates one barrier to effective assistance, which is distance. Doctors in whatever location can have access to these women and offer real-time support, especially in situations where it is either impractical or impossible for these women to go to the hospitals. States such as Arkansas and Virginia already operate a model that is similar to this. Their models have shown a remarkable impact in the number of deaths associated with pregnancies.

Also, certain other states are contributing by offering Medicaid reimbursements for midwives. This automatically increases the workforce available in the medical sectors. It had been noted earlier that the provision of midwives and doulas could positively impact maternal death rates significantly. It is thus impressive to see that some states are already implementing these strategies. This also gives the assurance that this suggestion works. Thus, if this action plan that is mostly implemented at state levels is implemented nationwide, the fruits will thus be universal. This is because the availability of more midwives would mean that patients will potentially have access to better healthcare. Deaths that result from the unavailability of a doctor or midwife would then be eliminated.

Finally, some states are taking steps to address the mental health challenges posed by childbirth. Missouri, for instance, is taking steps to address challenges related to not only physical health, but also the mental health of black mothers. It is unarguable that the mental state of a mother soon after birth can have potential consequences not just for the mother but for the child as well. Also, there is a high rate of suicide by new mothers, much to the point of being of concern to health experts.

It is also important to point out that substance abuse has been identified to be of significant impact both for pregnant mothers and new moms. It is also true that the rate of substance abuse is higher in the black community, making it an issue of priority. Hence, the steps taken by the state of Missouri is not only commendable but is worthy of emulation. The state has passed a bill that provides mental health treatments for

Medicaid-eligible mothers for more than a year after childbirth. This makes sure that the new mother has all the help and support she needs through this trying phase.

# CONCLUSION

It is true that high profile cases of disparities in the treatment of women in the black community, such as that of Serena Williams, has raised awareness about how racism, and other factors affect outcomes for black women, there is more that needs to be done. The scourge of racism will not be eliminated in a few years that would be a tall order for anyone to achieve. For real change to become visible, every sector involved in the provision of care for pregnant women of color needs to be responsive and decisive to be effective. If we, as a sovereign nation cannot adhere to the research and common-sense approaches to remedy the problems outlined in this book, it is indeed our fault!

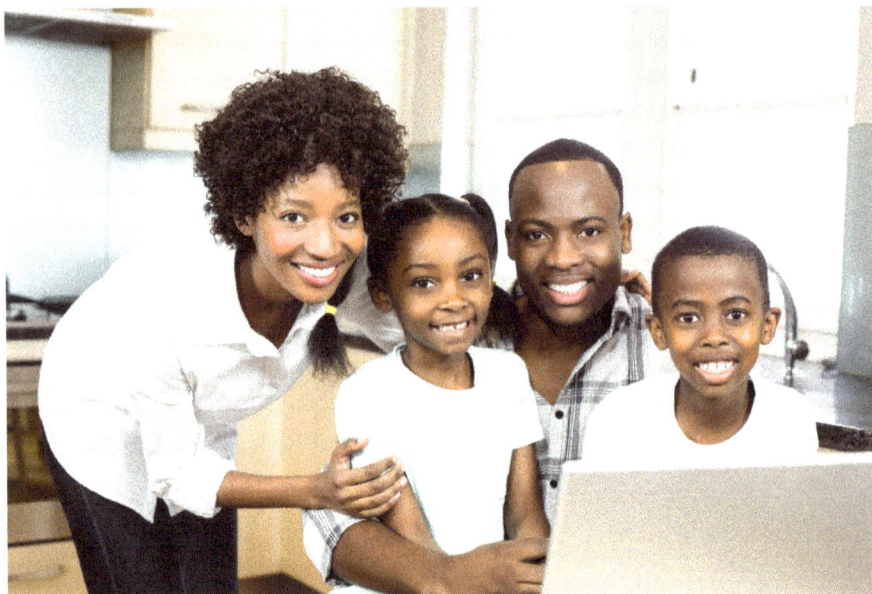
Baby and Family a great combination.

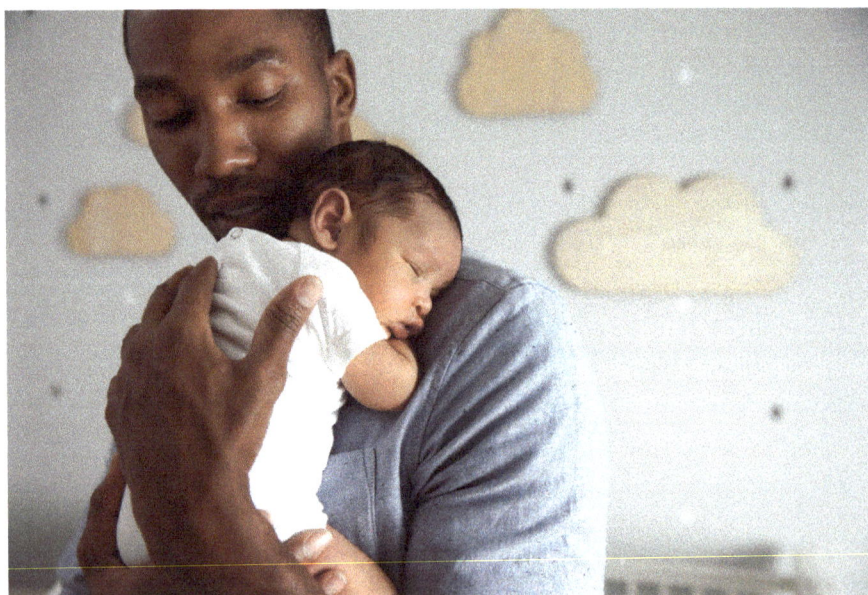
Baby and father can warm the heart!

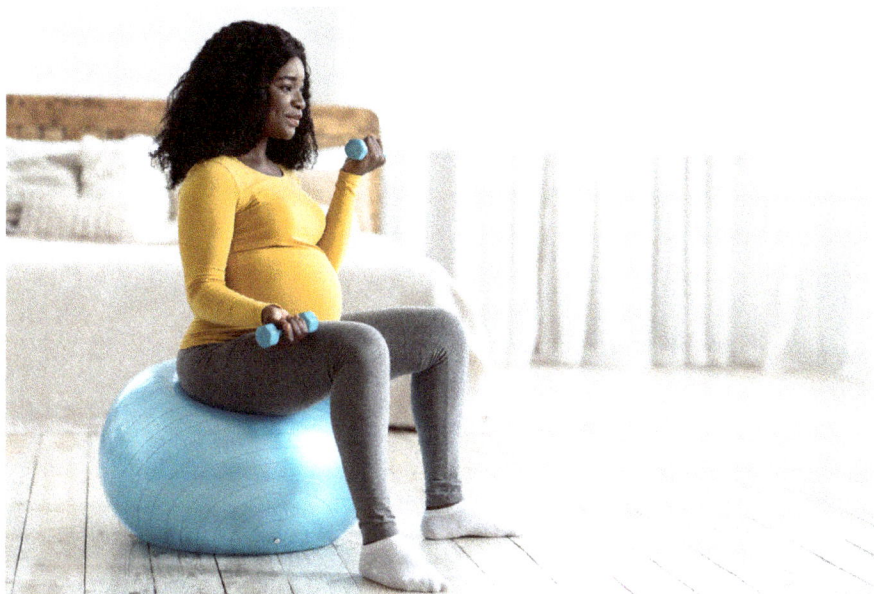

Pregnant mothers must get exercise regularly.

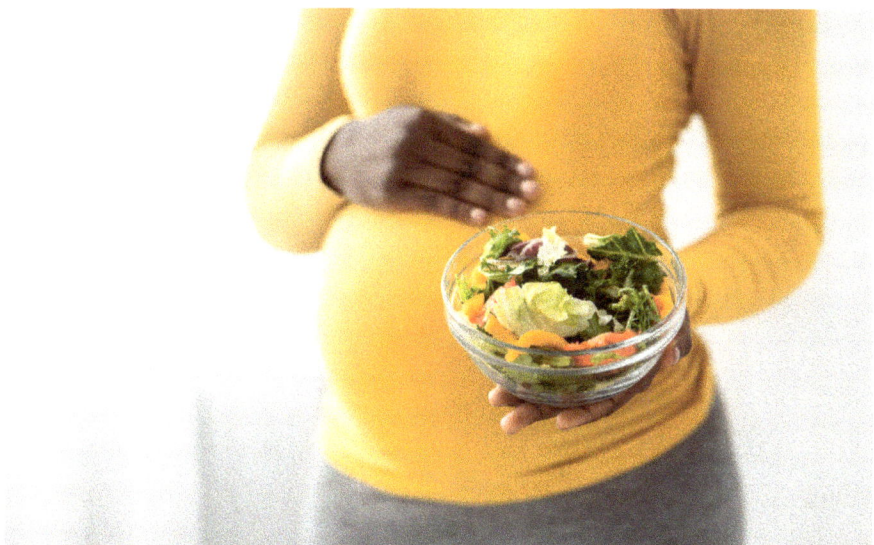

A proper diet is required for the health of an unborn child; remember:
When mom eats the unborn child eats.

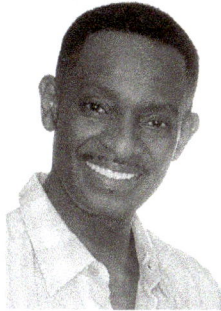

# BIO FOR STANLEY G BUFORD, PH.D.

In a previous book, directed to those who take parenting seriously in the Urban Centers of America; Former President Barrack Obama remarked: "Thank you for your interesting book on parenting."

Stanley G. Buford was born in Chicago, Illinois. He studied at Illinois State University and holds master's degrees from National-Louis University in Management/Human Resource Development and DePaul University in Curriculum Development. He recently completed work for a Ph.D. in Christian Education Leadership. The book you now hold represents the fruit of that labor with regards to his research/dissertation. He has also worked as a "results driven" teacher in Chicago Public Schools, the Archdioceses of Chicago and as a Charter School Employee.

Stanley has appeared as a guest on the nationally televised show, "Heartbeat of America," in a frank discussion concerning challenges to climbing corporate and educational ladders. He owns and operates a state certified management consulting business, Terkat Consultants Inc. He has been quoted in news articles, while lecturing at schools such as Northwestern, DePaul and the University of Illinois, on a variety of contemporary issues. An avid marathoner, actor, playwright and visionary.

Stanley has served as the Program Director of the School Partnerships Program, a school improvement project at DePaul University. He has also served as an adjunct faculty member at Concordia University. He founded his mentoring program, From Boys to Men Network Foundation, in 1991, to improve the quality of life for school-age boys in Chicago's inner city. In this non-fiction book, **Our Fault: The Infant Mortality Rate and the Black Community**, will enrich all readers and stakeholders concerned with the scourge of a high infant mortality for Black mothers in the United States. This work is a follow-up to his Amazon.com bestseller*: **Not All Teachers Are Parents, but All Parents Are Teachers!**

# REFERENCES

Bahadu, N. (2019, October 31) *8 ways we can actually reduce Black Maternal Mortality.* Retrieved from https://www.self.com/story/how-to-reduce-black-maternal-mortality.

Galvin G. (2019, August 1). *Black Babies Face Double Risks of Dying Before their First Birthday.* Retrieved from https://www.usnews.com/news/healthiest-communities/articles/2019-08-01/black-babies-at-highest-risk-of-infant-mortality.

Kliff, A. (2018, January 8). *American kids are 70 percent more likely to die before adulthood than kids in other rich countries. Retrieved* from https://www.vox.com/health-care/2018/1/8/16863656/childhood-mortality-united-states.

Lee, A. (1960) Maternal Mortality in the United States. *Phylon Journal. 38.* (3) 259 – 266. https://www.jstor.org/stable/274588?read-now=1&seq=1

Novoa, C. (2018, February 1*) Exploring African Americans' High Maternal and Infant Death Rates. Retrieved* from https://www.americanprogress.org/issues/early-childhood/reports/2018/02/01/445576/exploring-african-americans-high-maternal-infant-death-rates/#:~:text=Studies%20show%20that%20once%20African,with%20lower%2Dquality%20prenatal%20care.

Ogundimu, T. and Burns A. (2019, February 14) *Three Strategies that reduce infant mortality – and one that does not.* Retrieved from https://www.advisory.com/research/care-transformation-center/care-transformation-center-blog/2019/02/infant-mortality

Owens, D. and Fett S. (2019) Black maternal and infant Health: Historical legacies of slavery. *AJPH. 109.* (10) 1342-1345. https://ajph. aphapublications.org/doi/pdf/10.2105/AJPH.2019.305243

Roeder, A. (2019) *America is Failing its Black Mothers.* Retrieved from https://www.hsph.harvard.edu/magazine/magazine_article/america-is-failing-its-black-mothers/#:~:text=According%20to%20the%20U.S.%20Agency,women%2C%20and%20also%20more%20severe.

Taylor, J. Novoa, C. and Hamm, K. (2019, May 2), *Eliminating Racial Disparities in Maternal and Infant Mortality.* Retrieved from https://www.americanprogress.org/issues/women/reports/2019/05/02/469186/eliminating-racial-disparities-maternal-infant-mortality/

Villarosa, L. (2018, April 11). *Why America's Black Mothers and Babies are in a Life-or-Death Crisis.* Retrieved from https://www.nytimes.com/2018/04/11/magazine/black-mothers-babies-death-maternal-mortality.html?smid=tw-share

# NOTES

# NOTES

# NOTES

# NOTES

# NOTES

# NOTES

# NOTES

# NOTES

NOTES

NOTES